Mantle Cell Lymphoma:
Fast Focus Study Guide

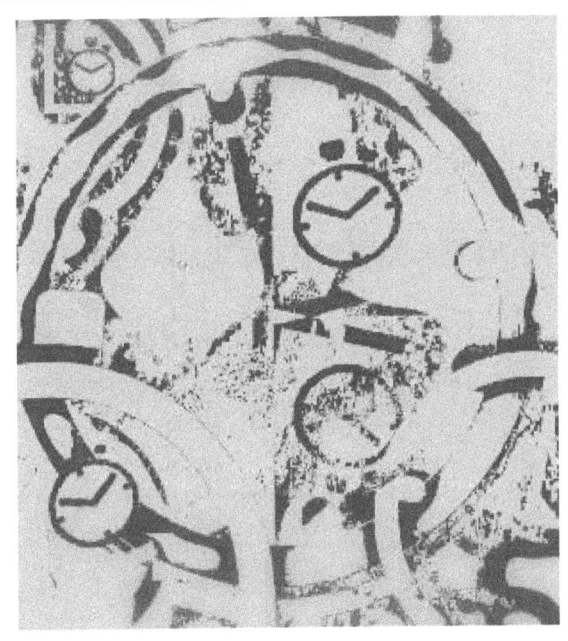

Acknowledgements

I dedicate this book to my beautiful wife and children, who I love more than all the water in all the oceans and all the seas.

CONTENTS

- This book is written for anyone who wants to learn more about Mantle Cell Lymphoma

- Put this book in your bathroom or on your coffee table.

- This is perfect for medical students, residents or physicians.

- This Fast Focus Study Guide will provide you with a practical review of the key information you need to know.

- Buy this book now if you want this quick and concise information

About 90% of patients with Mantle Cell Lymphoma will have stage IV disease at diagnosis. This lymphoma is known to cause an unusual condition known as lymphomatous polyposis.

Mantle cell lymphoma has some morphologic and clinical characteristics that are similar to CLL/SLL, so it is important to be able to tell these apart. Mantle cell generally is associated with a worse prognosis, and the treatment of these lymphomas is different.

Mantle cell lymphoma often presents with advanced disease characterized by circulating tumor cells. Diffuse adenopathy will be present in 70% to 90% of patients at the time of diagnosis.

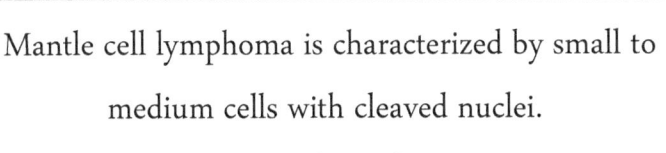

Mantle cell lymphoma is characterized by small to medium cells with cleaved nuclei.

Immunophenotype analysis shows FMC7+, sIg+, CD19+, CD20+, CD23-, CD5++, CD10-.

CLL will expresses CD23 and mantle cell lymphoma will not. CLL will not have FMC7 and shows only a dim expression of CD20 and dim surface immunoglobulin (sIg) expression. Mantle cell lymphoma will usually expresses bright CD20 and bright to moderate sIg, lacks CD23, and is FMC7+.

Mantle cell expression of cyclin D1 is unique
among lymphomas.

Mantle cell lymphoma is not terribly common. It accounts for about 6% of Non-Hodgkin lymphoma cases.

This disease involves men about 70% of the time with a male to female ratio of about 4:1.

The median survival times can vary, but overall these estimated as approaching 6 years for new patients.

We know that there is a survival variability among patients with Mantle cell lymphoma with some patients doing well and some patients doing quite poorly. We can now separate these patients into 3 groups: Indolent: Aggressive: and Very Aggressive.

Indolent mantle cell lymphoma accounts for about 15-20% of cases. These patients typically have a hypermutated IGHV, Low Ki-67 <10%, and lack of Sox-11.

Aggressive mantle cell lymphoma accounts for about 60-70% of cases. These patients typically have a Ki-67 of 10-30%, and lack are positive for Sox-11.

Highly aggressive mantle cell lymphoma accounts for about 5-15% of cases. These patients typically are characterized as blastoid. The have a Ki-67 >30%, and are characterized as positive for TP53, P16. The P16 abnormality is also known as cyclin dependent kinase inhibitor 2A (CDKN2A).

The prognosis is typically worse when the patient is found to have an un-mutated IGHV.

About 90% of mantle cell lymphomas will have extra nodal involvement. The most common locations of extra nodal involvement will include the bone marrow and the GI tract.

The most common cytogenetic abnormality in mantle cell lymphoma is the t (11:14) chromosomal translocation.

Extra nodal disease in the form of gastrointestinal involvement (lymphomatous polyposis) is common and has been reported in up to 80% of cases in some series.

Mantle cell lymphoma with hypermutated ighv has a better prognosis.

The Mantle Cell Lymphoma International Prognostic Index (MIPI) was developed to help estimate prognosis based on based on 4 independent prognostic factors: age, performance status, lactate dehydrogenase (LDH), and leukocyte count. Using the MIPI, patients were classified into low risk (44% of patients, median OS not reached), intermediate risk (35%, 51 months), and high risk groups (21%, 29 months).

The upfront treatment of newly diagnosed mantle cell lymphoma is primarily dependent on age and performance status.

Younger patients/patients with a good performance status are treated with regimens that included ARA-C. If the patient is not going to be taken to transplant then the possible treatments would include R-Hyper-CVAD/RMtx with ARA-C. If the patient is going to transplant then the regimen would still include ARA-C and would be something like RCHOP/RDHAP followed by ASCT.

In elderly or unfit patients, the treatment of choice is R-CHOP with maintenance rituximab. Alternative regimens would include R-Bendamustine with maintenance Rotuman.

Other options for patients that will not
tolerate R-CHOP or those with recurrent
disease include Bortezomib, Lenalidomide,
and ibrutinib.

Bortezomib as single agent for mantle cell

lymphoma has an overall response rate

30%

Lenalidomide was approved in patients who received at least 2 previous regimens and has response rate of about 28%. The CR rate was only 8%.

Ibrutinib was approved in patients relapsed mantle cell lymphoma after at least one previous treatment. The overall response rate was 67%.

This concludes Mantle Cell Lymphoma: Fast Focus Study Guide

Search Amazon Kindle books to find other study guides written by

JT Thomas, MD

Internal Medicine Study Guide

Hematology Study Guide

Medical Oncology Study Guide

Cardiology Study Guide